Alkaline Diet

Ultimate Alkaline Diet Guide To Improve Your Health
And Shed Pounds With Easy Alkaline Recipes

(The Key To A Healthy Lifestyle Is Alkaline Foods)

Joachim Kazmierczak

TABLE OF CONTENT

Introduction

Much has been written about the advantages of an alkaline diet in popular literature and on numerous websites. This essay is an attempt to find a balance between the evidence found in the sentfs literature. Life on earth is dependent on abnormal rH levels in and around living cells and organs. Human life requires a serum pH level of approximately 7.8

From the hunter-gatherer era to the present, there have been significant changes in the rH and net acid load of the human diet With the agricultural revolution (the last 2 0,000 years) and industrialization (the last 200 years), the ratio of potassium (K) to sodium (Na) and chlorine (Cl) to bsarbonate in the diet has decreased and increased, respectively. The ratio of rotaum to odum has been inverted; K/Na rrevoulu was 2 0 to 2 , while the modern det has a ratio of 2 to 6 . As compared to the pre-agricultural era, it is commonly believed that agricultural humans today consume a diet rich in magneum and rotaum, as well as fibre and saturated fat, added sugars, iodine, and chloride. This results in a diet that may induce metabolic acidosis consistent with genetically determined nutritional needs.

There is a gradual decline in renal acid-base regulator function with ageing, resulting in an increase in diet-induced metabolic acidosis in the modern diet. A low-carbohydrate, high-protein diet with an increased acid load causes very little change in blood chemistry and pH, but numerous changes in urinalysis. Amazingly, the human body is able to maintain a constant rH level in the blood, with the main compensatory mechanisms being renal and respiratory. The majority of the membranes in our bodies require an acidic rH to protect us and aid in digestion. It's been suggested that an alkaline diet can prevent a number of diseases and lead to significant health benefits.

Given that rhorhate is beneficial to bone health and results in a positive salsum

3

balance, there does not appear to be sufficient evidence to suggest that milk or cheese may be as detrimental as suggested. However, an additional mechanism by which the alkaline diet may improve bone health is the increase in growth hormone and the resulting effect on osteocalcin. There is some evidence that the K/Na ratio is significant and that excessive salt intake is detrimental. Even some governments are requiring the food industry to reduce the sodium content of our diet. In addition to affecting bone health, a high-protein diet may also be necessary for good bone health. Muscle wasting, however, appears to be reversed by an alkaline diet, and back pain may also benefit. Some chemotherapeutic agents may be more effective in an alkaline environment, but not others.

Is an Alkaline Diet Beneficial to Bone Health?

Numerous studies on the alkaline diet have utilised observational methods. Currently, these investigations have produced inconclusive results. On the other hand, observational research cannot provide conclusive answers. A correlation may be inferred from an observation. It demonstrates nothing.

Take a step back and consider the situation. 10 2 Observational study findings have been replicated in randomised clinical trials as a result of research into observational study methodology (a superior study design.) None of the 10 2 results from a randomised clinical trial held up!

The next logical step is to apply this concept to the alkaline diet and bone health. Multiple observational studies suggest that an alkaline diet may contribute to the development of strong bones. It is possible, however, that this is simply a series of chance encounters. Research that relies solely on participant observations disregards all other potential coincidences. For instance, they may all adhere to an alkaline diet and have strong bones.

Few randomised human studies on the association between an alkaline diet and bone health supported the contradictory findings of observational research. Here is what we've discovered:

The relationship between net acid excretion and calcium levels in urine is linear.

Calcium levels in the body and bone metabolism, as well as net acid excretion, are unrelated.

These findings suggest that the more acidic a meal is, the more calcium is excreted in the urine. Calcium levels in the body and bones are unrelated to calcium excretion through urine.

On one hand, an alkaline diet encourages the consumption of a wider variety of fresh fruits and vegetables. Increasing your consumption of fruits and vegetables is generally beneficial. On the other hand, the alkaline diet restricts protein consumption due to this food's acid-forming properties. Protein deficiency compromises bone health and should therefore never be avoided.

Chapter 1 : Atkins Phase Prior To Maintenance

The pre maintenance phase of the diet plan follows the orientation and OWL phases. This phase serves as the foundation for a balanced and healthy lifestyle in the foreseeable future. If you are within five to ten pounds of your target weight, you should do this. Although the process of weight loss would be slowed, you would acquire strategies that would ultimately assist you in achieving greater results. In the OWL phase, you would gradually increase your carbohydrate intake by 10 grammes per week. Once the maintenance week began, this increment would be increased to 2 0 grammes per week. Slowly, grammes of carbohydrates are added until you begin to lose weight.

During the period preceding maintenance, it is typical to lose less than one pound per week. According to the Atkins diet plan book, you should remain in this state until you reach your ideal weight and have maintained it for at least one month. The duration of this procedure is between one and three months. The objective is to reach "carbohydrate equilibrium," the point at which your carbohydrate intake is optimal and will support long-term weight maintenance. You can eat a variety of foods at this time; you can introduce new foods gradually while simultaneously increasing your carbohydrate intake at the correct rate. The recommended increase in carbohydrate consumption per week is 2 0 grammes. In this manner, the ideal weight could be maintained. Before adding a portion of a new food to a diet webpage or book, it is necessary to consult the carbohydrate counter. A half apple, half a cup of plain oats, a quarter cup of potatoes, and a third cup of beans all contain 2 0 grammes of cabs. This food is to be consumed daily and gradually increased as the weeks progress. The pre-maintenance process is not fully developed. It requires a delicate balance of exercise and carbohydrate counting in order to prevent further weight gain after a loss. It is essential to take the necessary precautions to monitor your carbohydrate consumption in order to prevent weight gain. The distinction between weight gain, loss, and maintenance is unclear. During pre-maintenance, you should be on the lookout for this very fine line. If consuming more carbohydrates does not prevent weight loss, metabolic resistance is likely high. Intensified exercise can be beneficial in this circumstance. Divide your weekly carbohydrate intake so that you consume a little less on a few days by eating a piece of fruit or a serving of sweet potatoes. The alternative method involves using the amount of carbohydrates saved to determine the days when you can enjoy yourself. Care should be taken to prevent a return of carbohydrate cravings, but if the pre-maintenance phase is followed correctly, long-term success is assured. It would help maintain weight and provide a balanced carbohydrate intake.

Youngster on Diets

Since the beginning of time, there have been the most obese children and adolescents in the twenty-first century. For safety reasons, due to the fast food and coffee shop culture, many parents choose to keep their children at home, which makes them even more sedentary and lethargic, eventually transforming them into couch potatoes who can spend countless hours watching television or computers together. Today's adolescents almost always spend the majority of their time on the phone or in front of televisions and computers, rather than engaging in activities that improve their health and well-being. As a result, they have become unfit, ill, and apathetic. In addition, it had a lasting impact on their nutrition, physical activity, and eating habits. Numerous games that were created with this in mind have been released. Providing the adolescents with some form of exercise within the walls. In this way, the Play Station 2's Dance Party Revolution and the new Nintendo Wii game system distinguished themselves in the market. They are an enjoyable form of exercise. Teens prefer it more. These games allow users to become completely immersed in the experience. As opposed to the static video games that were previously played there. This promotes the children's participation and is thus equally essential. Adults adore it because it's a great stress reliever and workout. "Jack becomes a dull boy when he works constantly." This adage is unquestionably true. Children and adolescents must be encouraged to engage in physical activity and explore the outdoors in this environment that is continuously expanding and enhancing. Teens learn from their experiences, and whether or not they admit it, they genuinely enjoy attending family-friendly events. Therefore, these activities must be encouraged. Plan family vacations that include activities such as mountain climbing, wall climbing, biking, hiking, and boating. You can also organise weekend camps or enrol in classes to learn a brand-new sport or hobby. Any activity the adolescent chooses to pursue must be supported in order to prevent falling behind. You may also encourage your adolescent or younger child to join a club for any sport they enjoy. They can participate in sports they are already familiar with or try a new one that piques their interest. Family games of softball, volleyball, or soccer are also highly recommended.

Chapter 2: Does the alkaline diet function?

Some individuals argue that the alkaline diet makes the body less acidic and more alkaline. Proponents of the diet claim that it promotes weight loss and combats disease. However, there is no evidence to support this claim. Some research indicates that following an alkaline diet may improve the health of individuals with kidney disease. However, this is not accomplished by altering blood rH. Instead, the alkalne diet encourages individuals to consume more fruits and vegetables and less processed meats and high-fat dairy products. For this reason, an alkaline diet may continue to promote health. A few studies indicate that consuming low-sugar foods improves health, even though they do not affect blood rH levels. In this article, we examine the myths surrounding the alkaline diet, whether they are true, and how the alkaline diet's foods can improve health.

Chapter 3: Does It Work?

What manu reorle believes is the primary advantage of an alkaline diet is false. The alkaline diet promotes the myth that it is difficult to change blood type with diet. This is false, and significant changes in blood rH can even be fatal. Diet is capable of altering the pH of urine and saliva. When the pH of these fluids changes, however, the rH of blood remains unchanged. Alkalinity indicates that something has a rH value greater than 7. The blood pH of the human body is approximately 7.8 ; the human body is naturally alkaline. The tomash is solid, allowing it to digest food. The pH of saliva and urine varies based on diet, metabolic rate, and other factors. Some research explains how sanser sell become more rare in an arid environment. Based on this research, proponents of the alkaline diet argue that a high rH level in the blood could prevent cancer. However, studies on alkalinity and sanser have involved sanser cells in a petri dish and not the human body. The foods consumed on this diet can, however, contribute to a healthy body weight. Doing so may prevent weight-related health problems such as diabetes.

Chapter 4: What causes a body to be acidic?

It's quite normal for our bodies to produce a variety of toxins throughout the day, such as when we breathe, eat, exercise, talk, and mrlu simply 'live' - as well as those produced by other types of metabolic reactions. The body neutralises them before moving on to other activities, so they do not cause any problems.

However, if you are living an unhealthy lifestyle, consuming acid-forming foods, or even suffering from a serious health condition such as kidney or liver failure, these levels can rise to unforgivable levels, leading to everything from minor health issues to life-threatening acidosis.

Your Eating Addiction

There are many things that can damage an elderly person's body and lead to degenerative diseases, but diet is without a doubt the worst offender, particularly the modern SAD or tandard American diet that many people follow. These highly processed and high-saturated fat foods are not only bad for your waistline, your mood, your skin, and your energy levels, but they can also create an environment in which bacteria, fungi, and viruses can thrive. Det is not the only criminal on the list. In the end, you can eat all the right kinds of food, but if you don't treat your body well and pay attention to your lifestyle, you will still have difficulty reducing acidity.

Other contributors to an asd's physique include:

Not enough sleep

When you burn the candle at both ends, your body misses a vital opportunity to repair, rejuvenate, and eliminate toxins accumulated throughout the day. If you don't get enough sleep, you're not giving your body the support it needs to rebalance and achieve an alkaline state.

Consuming alcohol

Alcohol poses two problems to the human body. Alsohol is a toxin that causes stress on the body's organs, such as the liver and the kidneys, which inhibits the body's natural pH neutralisation process and leads to the accumulation of toxins. Second, alcohol actually causes the production of stomach acid, resulting in both internal problems such as ulcers and a high acidity level throughout the body.

Extreme levels of stress are fatal. In response to a perceived threat, your body will release large quantities of the stress hormones cortisol and noradrenaline. In the past, these hormones would have helped us physically evade danger, whereas today it is primarily psychological and emotional factors that influence our behaviour. From the outside, this may not seem to easy make much of a difference, but on the inside, it's a very different story. These hormones won't be able to be expelled through renal action, so they will remain in our bodies, accumulate in our tissues, and increase our overall acid load, bringing our rH to a dangerous level. levels.

After a brief period of time, tre astuallu transforms into vsou cycle of acidity. Initial aspartame levels cause inflammation, and this inflammation causes illness, pain, and suffering. This in turn causes more stress, which in turn increases the acidity levels in the body and causes even more inflammation.

If you wish to learn more about inflammation and its effects on the body, my book, Natural Anti-Inflammatory Remedies, may be of assistance.

Food intoleranses

Food intolerance is your body's response to something you've eaten that isn't harmful. It attacks the food just like it would a foreign invader, with symptoms such as bloating, gas, diarrhoea, IBS, asthma, migraines, and more. When your body reacts in this manner, it places additional stress on your immune system and increases your body's adrenaline levels.

Over or under exersising

It's crucial to get the proper amount of exercise. Too little sodium causes our bodies to decline in health, slows down our bodily functions, causes us to gain weight, and prevents the body from producing normal levels of acidity and restoring balance effectively.

But don't force yourself to do excessive amounts of exercise, as this can be just as damaging. Any form of rhusal exercise increases lactic acid levels, which is the cause of the sore muscles you feel after exercising. When you exercise at an optimal level, your body reaps the benefits of the movement and processes waste in an efficient and effective manner. Just as with any other activity, mrrorer exercise is harmful; the body "struggles" to neutralise the asdtu level in the blood, and skne and shron's health conditions are frequently the result.

excessive intake of stimulants

You're feeling tired and frazzled and need a little boost to get you through the day, so you turn to coffee, tea, or even cigarettes to give you that boost. However, these things only serve to exacerbate your issues and push your body into deeper levels of addiction. The saffene in tea and coffee disturbs the hormonal balance, causing the release of more stress hormones into the bloodstream. The nicotine in cigarettes alters the reward centres in the brain and increases the levels of toxins in your bloodstream, resulting in increased anxiety, insomnia, and depression.

Medications

It has helped us overcome a multitude of health problems and live better, longer lives. But it comes with horrendous side effects, and to easy make matters worse, these medications are habit-forming and increase your risk of other diseases and health complications. It's hard to believe that such a large proportion of the world's population suffers from so many health problems when you consider how many of these acid-forming habits are on the rise. We are getting worse each year because we only treat the symptoms without addressing the root of the problem.

Chapter 5 : Does An Alkaline Diet

Rrevent Sanser?

The alkalne diet is one that has become popular in celebrity culture, with claims that it can help protect the body against diseases such as cancer and arthritis, as well as help you lose weight. The diet is able to test you for salmonella because it reduces the amount of salmonella in your body. The theory is based on the belief that salmon thrive in acidic environments and cannot survive in alkaline ones. Therefore, a "alkalizing diet" would promote a more alkaline environment in the body and prevent salmon from surviving. developing. Nonetheless, there are issues with Islam. The studies indicating that salmonella thrives in a toxic environment were conducted in a laboratory. Your body is very adept at maintaining its rH level without outside influence. It would be nearly impossible to change the sell environment in order to create a lean environment in our bodies. For example, the potato is extremely acidic, so we wouldn't want it to be more alkaline. Our asd-bae balance is well-regulated; blood rH is normally regulated by the body between 7.6 10 and 7.8 10 . If the rH level is too acidic or alkaline, this could be life-threatening and is an indication of a severe health issue, although it is not the underlying cause. Your body works hard to regulate and maintain the rH levels in your blood, making it difficult for you to alter these levels. Other areas of your body contain varying levels of aspartic acid, with your stomach containing the most in order to digest food. So even if you adhere to a strict alkaline diet, the results may not be what you expect. The diet does not encourage a person to eat healthily due to the fact that it contains unhealthy foods.

consuming more fruits and vegetables and avoiding processed foods helps with weight loss. However, it does not significantly affect the rH balance of your body.

Which foods are classified as alkaline and which are not?

In general, vegetables, fruits, and seeds are considered alkaline, whereas meat, beans, nuts, and grains are acidic. Therefore, an alkaline diet would consist primarily of vegetables and fruits, with minimal meat consumption. Eggs, dairy, and rose-colored foods are not considered alkaline and should be avoided on the diet. A diet focused on plant-based foods is similar to AICR's dietary recommendations for reducing the risk of cancer, with red meat limited to no more than 2 8 ounces per week. rer week, as well as avoiding rroseed meat. However, some truly healthy foods are classified as "side dishes," including whole grains, beans, and even some vegetables, such as sardines. Therefore, observe t mrle and adhere to AICR's New American Reduce your risk of heart disease by filling at least two-thirds of your plate with vegetables, fruits, and whole grains, and no more than one-third with meat, poultry, and fish.

Chapter 6 : Who Should Not Follow An Alkaline Diet?

Alkaline diets are generally healthy for those without a history of health issues; however, some individuals may experience hunger pangs or not consume enough protein to meet their needs. In addition to numerous harmful foods, certain nutritious foods are prohibited.

According to Tracy Lockwood Beckerman, RD, owner of Tracy Lockwood Nutrition in New York City, "some acidic foods, such as eggs and walnuts, are healthy." She warns that eliminating them can lead to compulsive behaviour and a departure from the nutrient-dense meals we require.

On the alkaline diet, which is not intended for weight loss, there are no portion control or exercise guidelines, which are recommended by the Centers for Disease Control and Prevention for disease prevention. In addition, you may experience hunger if you are unable to obtain sufficient protein from plant sources.

Function

Alkaline diets have been recommended for a variety of reasons, including weight loss, slowed ageing, and prevention of kidney stones, headaches, cancer, osteoporosis, and the common cold. However, the consumption of alkaline-ash foods has no effect on the pH of the body's tissues. Additionally, it is believed that alkaline diets boost energy levels.

Benefits

As alkaline fruits and vegetables contain fewer calories and fat than acidic meats, cereals, and dairy products, the majority of people who consume an alkaline diet will initially experience weight loss. Vegan and vegetarian diets may both benefit from alkaline diets. Thirdly, alkaline diets are typically more affordable than diets that include meat, dairy, and sweets.

Some individuals who have tried alkaline diets assert that they are more effective at regulating hunger than other weight-loss diets because the permitted meals are more filling due to their bulk and fibre content and there are no portion size restrictions.

Precautions

Before beginning any diet, cancer patients should discuss their dietary needs with a physician or dietitian.

If you have osteoporosis, arthritis, kidney stones, urinary tract infections, migraines, or any other ailment that an alkaline diet purportedly treats, you should not stop taking your medications.

Protein and calcium sources, such as lean meat and skim milk, which are permitted in moderation on other diets, are not permitted on an alkaline diet.

Alkaline diets are difficult for many individuals to follow, not only because of the limited food options, but also because eating out and living with relatives who do not adhere to the diet becomes more difficult. Due to the prohibition of processed foods, alkaline diets require additional time and effort to prepare meals.

Risks

A long-term alkaline diet may lead to nutritional deficiencies due to a lack of calcium, protein, and necessary fatty acids. In addition, individuals who stop taking prescription medications for conditions such as arthritis, cancer, diabetes, osteoporosis, or kidney stones because they believe an alkaline diet will suffice risk experiencing a worsening of their symptoms.

If dieters purchase alkaline water or other alkaline dietary supplements, they run the risk of being duped by companies that misbrand their products or easy make unsubstantiated health claims. In addition, the FDA asserts that certain samples of so-called alkaline water contain salmonella and other pathogens.

How easy is it to adhere to an alkaline diet?

The alkaline diet is difficult to adhere to.

Identify the acidic and alkaline foods. This can be a lot to remember. If you wish to feature alkaline-forming foods in your restaurant's menu, you will need to plan in advance.

Foods for an alkaline diet should be readily available.

A quick Google search yields an abundance of options, in addition to many books that can be purchased to provide even more options.

You may dine out while adhering to the alkaline diet, but be aware that some restaurants offer more pH-friendly dishes than others. If the menu features typical American cuisine, request a large salad with olive oil dressing and steamed vegetables instead of french fries or mashed potatoes. A Chinese buffet offers vegetable and egg-based soups, steamed broccoli, and sautéed chicken or tofu. Order chicken shish kebab instead of the acid-producing hummus and cheese pastry if you're going Greek.

You may be able to adhere to the alkaline diet if you plan in advance.

However, unless you hire someone to plan, shop for, and prepare your lunch and supper, there is no time savings associated with sticking to the diet. Using delivery services for meal kits is another way to save time on cooking.

There are available resources regarding alkaline diets.

Start with this book if you so choose.

This diet should not leave you feeling hungry.

Nutritionists place a high value on satisfaction, or the pleasant feeling of having eaten enough. Since there are so many fiber-rich, healthy grains and vegetables available, you should not feel hungry (and no-calorie limit).

Whether or not the Alkaline diet tastes good is solely your decision.

You easy make everything yourself, so you'll know who to blame if something doesn't taste good.

What type of exercise is recommended while on the Alkaline Diet?

Even though it is merely a method of eating, the Alkaline Diet does not prohibit exercise. Exercise reduces your risk of diabetes and heart disease, aids in weight loss, and increases your energy levels. On the majority of weekdays, doctors recommend 20 to 6 10 minutes of moderate-intensity activity, such as brisk walking.

To summarise

The alkaline diet encourages a high consumption of fruits, vegetables, and healthy plant foods, as opposed to processed junk food.

On the other hand, it is questionable whether the alkalizing properties of the diet contribute to the belief that it is healthy. No credible human studies exist to support these claims.

A small portion of the population may benefit in various ways, according to studies. A low-protein, alkaline diet may be beneficial for patients with chronic renal disease in particular.

Since the alkaline diet promotes whole, unprocessed foods, it is generally beneficial. There is no conclusive evidence that pH levels are involved.

Chapter 7: Dissecting the Relationship Between Alkaline Diet and Cancer

The body carefully regulates blood rH - how acidic or alkaline it is. Lungs, bones, and kidneys collaborate in a vital buffering system to keep blood acidity within a safe range.

A diet is neither acidic nor alkaline based on the pH of the foods. For example, it is not based on the consumption of acidic foods such as lemons and tomatoes. As foods are digested and metabolised, they create a more acidic or alkaline environment in the body. For example, animal protein is a major source of ulrhur-sontaining amino acids that increase the body's aspartate load. Vegetables and fruits are major sources of selenium and potassium, both of which can reduce insulin resistance.

An alkaline diet focuses on the need for the bodu to compensate for increased acid production as food is metabolised. It is unknown whether body adaptations to normal blood rH or small changes within the normal range have long-term effects. Could an acid- or alkaline-promoting diet alter the pH of the intracellular environment in ways that affect cell health and function?

Chapter 8: Instant Pot Cream Of

Broccoli Soup

Cream of Broccoli Sour is a comfort food, but making it in an Instant Pot makes it even better. This homemade our is ready to serve in less than thirty minutes and requires fewer than seven ingredients! Fresh broccoli, potatoes, leeks, and garlic give this dish a traditional flavour, but the addition of lemon garlic cashew cream gives it a smooth taste that you will enjoy. Plant-based, gluten-free, and dairy-free.

Ingredients

Soup
- 2 cup raw cashews soaked
- 2 cup water
- juice of 4 fresh lemon
- 2 teaspoon sea salt
- 2 teaspoon granulated garlic
- For topping 4 tablespoon toasted pistachios
- 8 cups fresh broccoli or frozen
- 16 cups vegetable broth
- 2 large russet potato peeled and chopped
- 2 leek chopped
- 12 cloves of garlic
- 2 teaspoon sea salt
- 1 teaspoon black pepper

Lemon Garlic Cashew Cream

Instructions

1. Add all soup ingredients to Instant Pot.
2. Easy cook on high pressure for 10 minutes.
3. Quick release pressure when soup is finished.
4. Allow soup to cool slightly.
5. Using small hand blender, blend a portion of soup vegetables to create a creamy texture.
6. Blend as much or little as you like, however more blending will result in a creamier soup with no vegetables.
7. Lemon Garlic Cashew Cream
8. Add all ingredients to high speed blender like Vltamix.
9. Blend until completely smooth.
10. Add cream to soup and stir slowly until all cream is absorbed into the soup.

11. Top with toasted pistachios.

Summer Squash Salad

Ingredients

- 4 tablespoon of extra virgin olive oil

- 2 teaspoon of smoked paprika

- 2 teaspoon of dried chives

- ¼   teaspoon of salt

- ½ of black pepper

- 2 1 tablespoon extra-virgin olive oil

- 4 teaspoon of salt

- 5-10 small yellow summer squash or green zucchini cut into small, flat pieces

- ¼ teaspoon of black pepper

- 4 cups of cherry tomatoes, halved

- 4 cups of tightly packed arugula

- 2 medium of avocado, pitted, peeled and diced

- 8 green onion, finely chopped

- Dressing

- Juice of 6 limes
  Instructions

1. You can easy make the squash on the grill or in the oven.

2. For the grill: toss the squash with 2 1 tablespoon of olive oil, 4 teaspoon of salt, and 1/2   teaspoon of pepper.

3. Easily put on kabob skewers and grill for about 20 minutes over medium heat, turning every 5-10 minutes or until slightly cooked through.

4. Remove from grill and allow to cool.

5. For the oven: Preheat the oven to 450º F. Toss the squash with 2 1 tablespoon of olive oil, 4 teaspoon of salt, and 1/2 teaspoon of pepper.

6. Roast the squash on a rimmed baking sheet for 45 to 50 minutes. Allow to cool.

7. Add the tomatoes, arugula, avocado, bell pepper, and green onion to a large bowl.

8. Add the squash once cool.

9. In a smaller bowl, whisk together the lime juice, olive oil, smoked paprika, chives, salt and pepper.

10. Pour the dressing over the salad and stir to combine.

11. Serve with your favorite protein

List of Ingredients:

- Olive oil: 2 Glug
- Garlic: 2 clove
- 1 lemon: Squeeze Juice
- Pink salt: 2 pinch

- Chickpeas (drained): 2 00g (Soak for one night)
- Almonds: 2 handful
- Tahini: 2 tbsp.
- Cumin: 2 pinch

Roll-Ups:

- Coriander/cilantro: 2 bunch
- Sliced capsicum (matchsticks): 2

- Zucchinieasy make : 4 medium
- Sliced Carrots (matchsticks): 2
- Sliced Cucumber (matchsticks): 2
- Avocado (remove skin and sliced): 2

Methods:

1. In the first step, easily put all the hummus ingredients into one food processor and process them to easy make a smooth blend.
2. You can increase the quantity of lemon and olive oil according to your preference.
3. Set the hummus aside.
4. Roll Ups for Alkaline Sushi.
5. Chop both ends of zucchini and peel it with the help of one vegetable peeler.
6. Easy make thin zucchini strips and spread one tablespoon of hummus on the strip.
7. Add some pieces of avocado, vegetables, and coriander to the hummus.
8. Sprinkle sesame seeds and roll up zucchini.
9. Sushi is ready to serve.

Cucumber Salad With Borage Flowers

Ingredients

2 cucumber - halved, seeded, and sliced
10 borage leaves
20 fresh borage flowers
4 tablespoons extra-virgin olive oil
2 tablespoon lime juice
salt and freshly ground black pepper to taste

Directions

1. Combine olive oil, lime juice, salt, and pepper in a bowl and stir together.
2. Add sliced cucumber, cover, and refrigerate for 2 hour.
3. Sprinkle with borage leaves and borage flowers just before serving, as the flowers wilt quickly.

Srisu Asian Noodle Salad

Ingredients

Dressing
- 1 cup raw almonds, chopped
- 8 tablespoons sesame oil
- 4 tablespoons Bragg Aminos
- ½ tablespoon hot chili oil

- 1 package thin Buckwheat Soba Noodles
- 1 cup green onion
- 20 pieces tofu (optional)
- 2 stalk celery, chopped
- 1 cup Mung bean sprouts
- 1 cup red pepper, chopped

Instructions

1.	Easy cook the noodles, drain, and rinse in cold water.

2.	Mix the Sesame oil, Bragg® Aminos, and hot chili oil.

3.	Add the dressing to the noodles and toss well.

4.	Cover and chill for several hours or overnight. Just prior

5.	to serving, stir in the vegetables, and top off with the almonds.

Raw Lemon Meltaway Balls

INGREDIENTS

- 4 teaspoons organic vanilla extract
- 1/2   cup organic coconut oil 2 1 cup almond flour
- 2 /6   cup organic raw coconut flour
- 1 teaspoon pink himalayan salt
- –1-5   tablespoon organic maple syrup
- 6 organic lemons

INSTRUCTIONS

1. Easily put all ingredients into a food processor and process until well combined.
2. Take out about a spoonful at a time and roll them in the palms of your hand into a ball shape.
3. Leave them plain or roll in shredded coconut flakes, almond flour, or powdered sugar (not raw).
4. Easily put them in the refrigerator to firm for about –35 to 40 minutes.
5. Keep them in the refrigerator until ready to serve because they will just get soft if left out at room temperature as the coconut oil melts.

Tasty Salad Made With Pasta

A three-quarter cupful of Sun-dried Tomatoes.

A quarter cupful of sliced Onions.

4 tbsp of Almond milk.

4 tbsp of Sea salt.

4 sprints of Cilantro.

2 and a half tbsp of Maple syrup.

4 tbsp of fresh Lime juice.

2 packet of Spelt penne.

25 Avocados cut in sizes.

½ cupful of Olive oil.

Procedures

Prepare the pasta according to the producer's instructions.

Combine all of the ingredients in a large mixing bowl.

Mix them very well and enjoy.

Homemade Vinaigrette

Ingredients:

- 4 teaspoons thyme, fresh
- 2 teaspoon oregano, dry
- 1 teaspoon sea salt
- ½ teaspoon cayenne pepper
- 12 tablespoons olive oil
- 4 tablespoons Seville orange juice
- ½ red onion medium, finely chopped
- ½   white onion medium, finely chopped
- 2 key lime, juiced

Instructions:

1. Finely chop the red and white onion.
2. In a mason jar or any other jar with a lid, squeeze the key lime, add the olive oil, Seville orange juice, finely chopped onion, thyme, oregano leaves, sea salt, and cayenne epper.
3. Alternatively, instead of using a mason jar, you can just put all the ingredients in a bowl and mix them with a whisk.
4. Taste and adjust flavor as needed, adding more key lime juice for acidity, or extra virgin olive oil for richness.
5. Close the lid and shake for a couple of seconds.

Cacao And Sesame Seed Smoothie

Ingredient
- 2 tablespoon vanilla extract
- 4 tablespoons raw cacao powder
- 2 frozen cauliflower piece
- 2 tablespoon sweetener made from monk fruit
- Optional cacao nibs on top
- 4 cups almond milk (homemade) (or any unsweetened plant milk)
- 4 tablespoons tahini butter
- 2 tablespoon of raw almond butter

Instructions
1. Blend all smoothie ingredients until smooth and creamy.
2. Adjust the flavor by adding more of any item to your liking.

The Brussels Sprouts Were Roasted.

Ingredients:

-1 teaspoon sea salt

1/2   teaspoon black pepper
-1-5 pounds Brussels sprouts, trimmed and halved

-6 tablespoons olive oil

Instructions:

Preheat oven to 450 degrees Fahrenheit.

In a large bowl, mix together the Brussels sprouts, olive oil, sea salt, and black pepper.

Transfer the mixture to a baking sheet and bake for 45 to 50 minutes, stirring once halfway through.

Enjoy as is or serve with your favorite dipping sauce!

Dredging Salad With Garlic

Ingredients:

½ teaspoon sea salt

½ teaspoon freshly ground black pepper

2 cup safflower oil

½ cup apple cider vinegar

4 teaspoons dry mustard

2 teaspoon garlic, minced

2 teaspoon paprika

Directions:

1. Easily put vinegar, mustard, garlic, paprika, salt, and pepper to taste, in a mixing bowl.

2. Add oil, beating with wire whisk.

3. Chill and serve over a favorite salad.

Sour Vegetables With Quinoa

Ingredients

16 cups vegetable broth

2 (2 10 ounce) can chickpeas, drained

1 cup quinoa

salt and ground black pepper to taste

2 1 cups frozen corn, thawed

2 avocado - peeled, pitted, and diced

6 tablespoons olive oil

6 medium onions, chopped

4 green bell peppers, chopped

2 carrot, diced

2 stalk celery, diced

12 cloves garlic, minced

6 tablespoons ground cumin

2 teaspoon chili powder

2 (28 ounce) can crushed tomatoes

20 green chile peppers, seeded and minced

Directions

1. Heat oil in a large stock pot over medium heat.
2. Stir in onions, bell peppers, carrot, celery, garlic, cumin, and chili powder. Cook until vegetables are tender, about 20 minutes.
3. Mix in crushed tomatoes and green chile peppers.
4. Pour in broth, chickpeas, and quinoa. Season with salt and pepper.
5. Bring to a boil; reduce heat to low and simmer for 60 minutes.
6. Mix corn into the soup until heated through, about 10 minutes.
7. Serve in bowls and top with avocado.

www.ingramcontent.com/pod-product-compliance
Lightning Source LLC
Chambersburg PA
CBHW060659030426
42337CB00017B/2701